YOGA FOR BACK PAIN

YOGA FOR BACK PAIN
A practical guide to healing

Emil J. Lewis

Yoga is the journey of the self, through the self, to the self.

The Bhagavad Gita

Índice

Introduction

With so many yoga books out there to choose from, it is sometimes difficult to find the right one for us, which solves a problem that is afflicting us, such as back pain. This book was written just for those who have a need and are looking for a solution.

Here you will not find endless chapters in which we talk about the history of yoga from a philosophical point of view, nor will we make distinctions between the different types of yoga or we will talk extensively about the benefits of this discipline on the body and mind of people.

This is a practical book. Those who buy it are looking for a solution to their problem, back pain, be it lumbar, cervical or another form. And this is what this book offers: practical solutions for back pain, using a series of yoga asanas, body mudras, relaxation and breathing exercises.

Each exercise or asana is explained in detail, but always from a very practical point of view. I will explain how to correctly perform each movement, how to breath properly during the practice and, of each asana, will be explained in detail the benefits (for the back and the rest of the body) and any potential contraindications. Each asana, however, is accompanied by illustrations that facilitate the understanding of the movements to be performed.

In addition to the asanas, the book also includes other types of exercises that, in combination with the asanas, help to loosen muscle tension, reduce stress (a non-secondary cause and almost always present in back pain, since it generates tension muscle that often concentrates in the lumbar and shoulder area) and in general to increase psycho-physical well-being.

These are relaxation exercises, which are often practiced at the beginning and end of a session of yoga, mudra (in this case, we will use body mudra) and pranayama, or breathing control exercises (or rather, of awareness of breathing).

Finally, in addition to presenting the various exercises, techniques and asanas individually, in this book you will also find sets of exercises for each type of back pain. In this way you can combine the exercises and the asanas that best lend themselves to your situation and get the maximum benefit from them.

From personal experience I can guarantee that the practice of yoga on a regular basis, together with relaxation exercises (very useful for reducing muscular tensions but also, and above all, mental stress), has been the solution I have been looking for years. Years of backache caused by endless hours sitting incorrectly in front of a screen, the accumulation of tension in the lumbar area, neck and shoulders and in general an inability to listen to my body, stop for a moment and take care of myself.

In addition, of course, to the stress that I had been accumulating for years, caused above all by the way in which I faced certain work situations or even personal situations.

In my case, all this produced two hernias at the lumbar vertebrae, which often caused great pain and limited me greatly in everyday life, to the point where I often had to help with my hands to get out of bed or not be able to tie my shoes alone.

But the fault, now I know, was mainly mine (not to say uniquely).

The body sends us signals continuously, both on a physical and mental level. Often we are not able to listen to him (or we do not want to do it) and this is why the body has to resort to extreme measures to make itself felt, just like pain or stress.

The signals were sent to me continuously, but I did not want to listen to them. Then the body (and the mind) could not help but "raise the voice". For my own good. This has meant going from small nuisances to intense pain, from a small and normal level of stress to suffering from a severe form of insomnia.

The yoga asanas and relaxation exercises that are proposed in this book have the primary benefit of reconnecting with our body and mind, to help us regain consciousness of the body and to be able to really perceive it again. This is the first step towards healing.

I therefore encourage you to take responsibility for your recovery, to learn to listen to the signals that your body sends you and to start this healing process that will give you back the quality of life you had lost.

Healing from back pain is not only possible, but it can also be a wonderful journey that will not only restore that lost elasticity, but also a renewed awareness of yourself.

Enjoy your trip.

Asana

In this chapter we will talk about yoga asanas. What they are, how they should be performed and what benefits they bring to our psycho-physical health.

We will also describe in detail thirty-seven asanas specifically selected for their beneficial effects on back pain. Each asana has been illustrated so as to facilitate understanding and execution.

What are asanas?

We define asanas (in Sanskrit आसन) the positions or postures that are used during the practice of yoga, with the aim of exercising a psychophysical benefit on body and mind.

The historical moment in which the populations of the Indian continent began to meditate using the postures we know today as asanas is not exactly known.

The first written reference to this term is found in the Yoga Sutra of Patanjali, a text dating back to the III century BC which contains a collection of 196 sutras (aphorisms) about yoga.

In these texts, Patanjali describes the techniques of body control through the mind, citing eight elements, including the asanas.

In Yoga Sutra Patanjali defined yoga as "calming the movements of the mind" and wrote about asanas that "the posture in yoga is stable and easy" (we will see in more detail the importance of this concept in the following paragraphs).

There is an indeterminate number of poses, some claim that more than a thousand, and the names of many of the asanas are inspired by the natural world (position of the cobra, the fish, the monkey, the tree, the mountain, etc.), although sometimes you can find slightly different names between one text and another.

According to the texts, it has been tried to classify the postures according to different categories such as how to perform them (standing posture, sitting, etc.) or the type of movement that takes place during the asana (push-ups, twists, balance, etc.).

In this book we will use the Sanskrit name of the asana and its most commonly accepted translation and we will focus on a specific set of positions whose main benefits are to restore the elasticity of the spine and eliminate or significantly reduce back pain, both in the lumbar area, cervical or anywhere else.

How to practice the asanas

Evidently, in order to get the most benefit from the asanas you will need to do them properly, especially by practicing without effort. In order to achieve this result it will be necessary to devote oneself to the practice of both asanas and breathing control techniques. For this reason, when the asanas are described, particular emphasis is placed on breathing.

The asanas, are postures that act through the movements of contraction and muscle lengthening, sometimes going beyond the normal limits of elasticity that are achieved in the usual positions that we assume during the day.

To achieve this result it is necessary to practice the asanas in a state of relaxation, both physical and mental, proceeding to the gradual and progressive stretching of the muscles, without straining (the absence of effort is a very important concept in yoga), otherwise the muscle, instead of lengthening, will tend to stiffen.

It is important to remember that the muscles are almost never fully stretched, so practicing the asanas seems to go beyond the normal limits of elasticity of your muscles, while in fact what you are doing is giving back to your body a capacity that it has been decreasing over the years (due to sedentary lifestyle or excessive sports, which has the consequence of reducing the ability to stretch muscles).

Taking a step back, let's now look at the basic elements in order to perform an asana correctly, starting with immobility.

As well as for muscle elasticity, which we have seen should be achieved progressively, the ability to maintain a long posture is a skill that also must be developed over time.

Keeping an asana over time requires practice, patience and knowledge of your body. It goes from maintaining a position just 1 or 2 minutes (as often happens during yoga classes for beginners), up to keep them for hours (this is a skill normally attributed only to very few Indian Yogins, who follow the sacred texts of yoga to the letter and have reached this level in years of practice).

The book indicates, according to the asanas, indicative durations to try to reach, often indicated by the duration of the breaths. It is important to remember that practicing yoga is not a competition (neither with oneself nor with other practitioners), but a quest to develop the ability to listen to one's body.

In addition to the ability to remain immobile during a certain period of time, it is equally important to develop the absence of effort, which as we have already said is a characteristic of yoga.

The absence of effort goes hand in hand with the absence of competition, as we have already said previously. Getting rid of this mental scheme can be difficult especially at the beginning for us Westerners, accustomed to living in a competitive society, which measures everything, that assigns a vote or a label to everything, but it is necessary to reach that state of tranquility that it will allow us to perform asanas in the absence of effort.

The concept of effortlessness should not, however, be confused. It does not mean not engaging, but rather not going beyond the limits of elasticity, stretching or normal contraction of the muscles. If we realize that, for example, our muscles are visibly vibrating during the practice of an asana, we are probably doing the position incorrectly.

All this obviously requires time, constant practice (better if daily) and the ability to let go of that competitive anxiety typical of modern society. It is important to always keep in mind that it is not a competition (not even with oneself), but it's about learning to know your body.

In support of the practice comes another fundamental resource of yoga: proper breathing. Breathing is in a sense the dynamic element within the static nature of the asanas in a yoga session, as well as the tool through which to learn about our body.

Already in ancient texts such as Patanjali's Yoga Sutra, breathing is indicated as a fundamental element to realize the body-mind union. It actually carries prana, which literally means "life" in Sanskrit (पुराण) and it is considered to be a subtle energy which all living beings are endowed with, in the body.

The control of breathing is therefore called pranayama (translatable as conscious breathing, from the Sanskrit *"prana"*, energy, and *"yama"*, control or expansion).

We will not go into this book in detail regarding pranayama and the various breathing control techniques, limiting ourselves to hinting (for those wishing to deepen this topic) that prana is in turn categorized or constituted by what the ancient texts call the five currents of prana, or *Pancha Vayu* (from the Sanskrit *"pancha"*, five, and *"vayu"*, air). These *vayus* are, respectively, *Prana, Apana, Samana, Udana* and *Vyana*, and can be understood as distinct manifestations of the energy of respiration.

Returning to the practice of asanas, we can simplify by recalling that breathing is composed of two main phases: inhalation and exhalation. The control of the rhythmicity of these two phases, the awareness of the movement of inhalation and exhalation, and therefore the ability to concentrate on breathing, is fundamental in the practice, since it will allow the relaxation of the muscles and their ability to lengthen them.

In the same way, by concentrating on breathing, we will be able to maintain the position required by the asana that we are performing, in the absence of effort and with total consciousness, listening to our body and mind.

Precisely the mind is the last (certainly not in terms of importance) element that we will discuss now in relation to the execution of the asanas. Until now we have mentioned physical elements such as immobility, the absence of effort and the focus on breathing, but in the practice of yoga, body and mind go hand in hand and are inseparable (after all, the same root of the term "yoga" refers to the verb "to unite").

The mind is the tool that allows us, among other things, to create the image (mental, precisely) of our body, through practice. The creation of this image, the perception of muscular bundles, of the joints, of the asymmetries that occur in our body, is fundamental in order to apply the postural corrections necessary in the practice of yoga.

However, during practice, the mind (whose nature is to be restless) will try to distract us with a multitude of thoughts, rebelling against the immobility of the body. Just as the absence of effort is a concept that we have seen must be applied on the physical plane, even on the mental level we must maintain the same attitude, in this case avoiding "trying" not to have thoughts (something almost impossible), but limiting ourselves to observe the mind and its activity, which will be reduced with assiduity in the practice of yoga, allowing us to reach a higher state of consciousness.

All this is directly related to the objectives of yoga practice and to the execution of the asanas, which allow to eliminate blockages and tensions on the physical level (often just in the torso area, with particular emphasis on the abdominal and back areas).

Although it may seem paradoxical, except in cases of undeniable pain, most people live in a state of unawareness, which leads to not recognizing these tensions or blockages.

As we have seen before, the observation of our body and the practice of asanas, causes these tensions to be brought back to a conscious level, thus allowing to recognize any physical problems and to resolve them with the stretching of the muscles and the exercises of relaxation.

General benefits of the asanas

Yoga postures have great physical and mental benefits, many of which have been proven by modern Western science. Among the main psycho-physical benefits we list:

- improve flexibility

- improve strength

- improve balance

- reduce symptoms of lower back pain

- improve the immune system

- regulation of blood pressure

- improve blood circulation

- regulation of sugar levels, cholesterol and triglycerides

- beneficial for asthma and chronic obstructive pulmonary disease (COPD)

- increase energy and decrease fatigue

- strength the cardiovascular system

- increase tissue oxygenation

- shorten labor and improve birth outcomes

- improve digestion

- reduce hypertension

- reduce weight

- reduce insomnia

- reduce stress and anxiety

- improve memory

- improve concentration

List of asanas

Below you will find a list (in alphabetical order) of thirty-seven asanas particularly indicated for back pain, cervical or lumbar pain. For each asana is indicated the starting position to be taken, the movements to be performed during the performance, the benefits for the back and the general ones for our health, as well as any contraindications.

Adityasana (pose of Aditi)

Starting position: sitting on the ground, legs bent forward, knees apart. Grasp the ankles, join the soles of the feet, the arms will be stretched and the shoulders pushed backwards.

Asana: flex the torso forward and at the same time move the hands from the ankles to the tip of the feet, overlapping them.

Before flexing the torso, lengthen the spine by inhaling and relaxing the shoulders while exhaling. After some repetitions you can finally move to the final asana, to keep for about a minute.

Benefits for the back: tones up the back muscles.

Other benefits: tones the genital system, preserving it in good health, increases sexual potential, eliminates headaches, stomach ache and menstrual pain in women.

<u>This asana, if performed in the menstrual period, increases its flow. It is therefore advisable to avoid it in case of abundant flow.</u>

Contraindications: with the exception of those concerning the abundant menstrual flow, none.

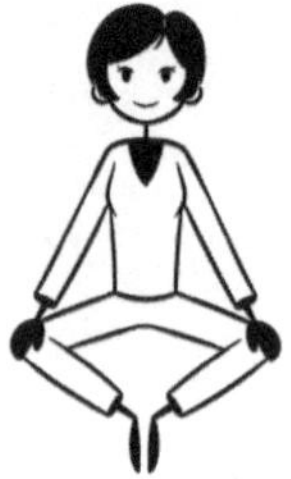 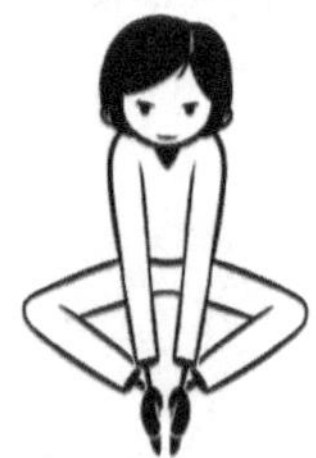 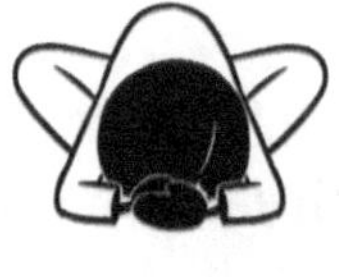

Anantasana (side-reclining leg lift pose)

Starting position: lying on the side, bending the inner forearm (the one closest to the floor) so that the hand can support the head (wrist on the temple, palm on the ear, fingers on the neck). The other arm is extended along the side.

Asana: bend the leg that is on top, resting the foot on the thigh of the other leg. Grasp the ankle with the corresponding hand and stretch the leg upward.

Hold the position for different breaths (5 to 20), then change sides.

Benefits for the back: relaxes the back and eliminates the pain.

Other benefits: prevents the formation of inguinal hernias, articulates the joint and elasticizes the muscles.

Contraindications: none.

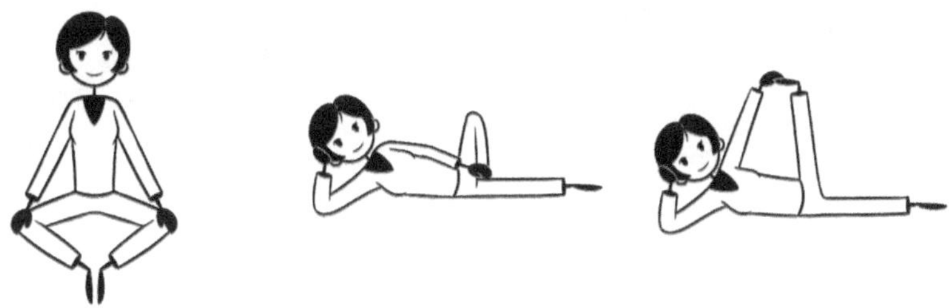

Anjaneyasana (low lunge pose)

Starting position: kneel, inhale. Bring one foot forward, exhaling, keeping the leg bent. The leg in the strict sense (ie the part below the knee) should be parallel to the thigh (upper part of the knee) of the other leg (intended as the lower limb).

Asana: breathing deeply, stretch your arms above your head, looking up. Exhale. Stay in this position for 10 breaths, then inhale and then, slowly exhaling, lower the arms and sit on the heels.

Benefits for the back: elasticizes the vertebral column, tones the whole skeleton.

Other benefits: improves the respiratory capacity, slims the hips, strengthens the pelvis.

Contraindications: none.

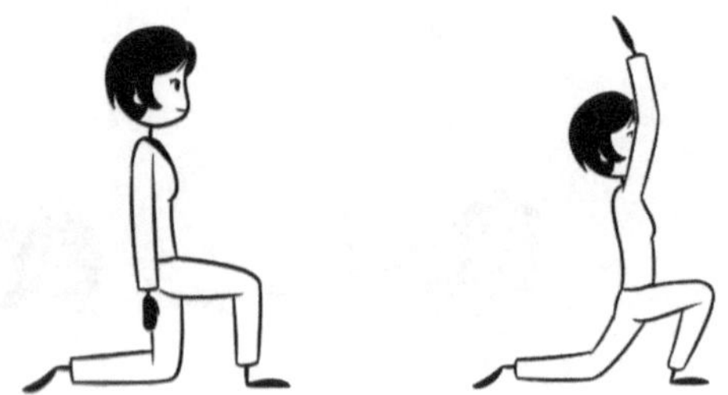

Ardha Bhujangasana (half cobra pose)

Starting position: sitting on the heels, inhaling, raising on the knees; exhale, bring a foot forward, so that a right angle between thigh and leg is formed and that the leg is parallel to the thigh.

Asana: inhale deeply and, exhaling, bring the body forward, reducing the angle between the thigh and the leg and increasing the angle behind the other limb.

Keep your torso straight, open your shoulders and relax your arms. Hold the position for 10-20 breaths.

Inhaling deeply, bring the body back. Exhale, return sitting on the heels.

Benefits for the back: elasticizes the skeleton.

Other benefits: improves the sense of balance, prevents and dissolves the fat formations around the hips.

Contraindications: none.

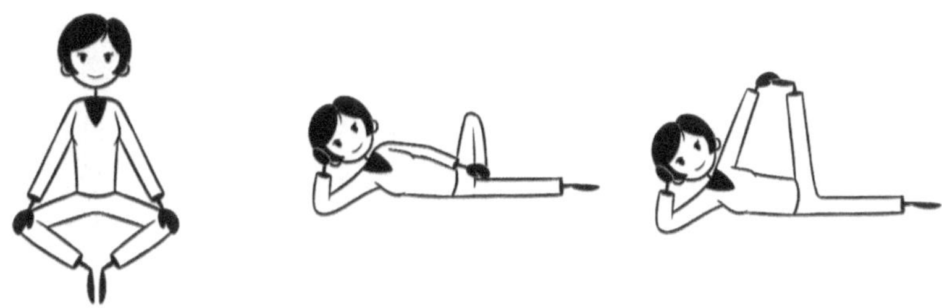

Ardha Chandrasana (half-moon pose)

Starting position: sitting on the heels. Inhaling, kneeling, so as to form a right angle between thighs and legs. Exhale, extend a leg sideways, with the sole of the foot resting on the ground. Inhaling, raise the arms open sideways.

Asana: exhaling, slowly flex the torso on the side of the extended leg. The corresponding hand rests with the back on the thigh or on the knee. The opposite arm forms an extension of the hip and surrounds the head.

Hold the position for 5-10 breaths. Breathing in, lift the bust up; exhale, bring down your arms.

Inhale again and, exhaling, return sitting on your heels. Repeat the exercise on the other side, with the same execution methods.

Benefits for the back: strengthens the muscles of the bust.

Other benefits: slims the hips and makes the body agile.

Contraindications: none.

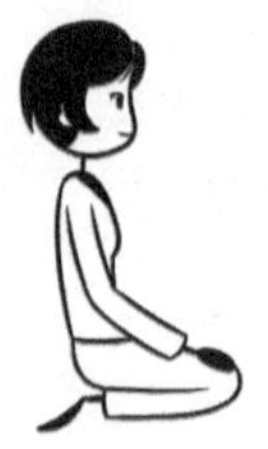 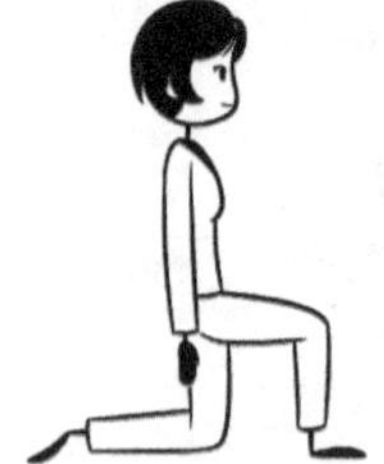 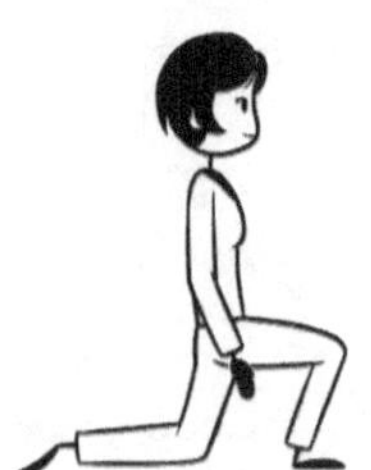

Ardha Natyasana (half dance pose)

Starting position: standing, upright torso, legs stretched out and feet together. Interlock the fingers with your hands, palms facing down and arms outstretched.

Asana: breathing slowly, bring your arms up, over your head. Exhale, arch your neck backwards and watch your fingers while keeping your arms straight.

Maintain the position from 5 to 20 breaths. Inhale, stretch all the muscles, exhale, untwist your fingers and bring your arms slowly along your sides.

Benefits for the back: tones the spine.

Other benefits: strengthens all the muscles and straightens the rounded shoulders.

Contraindications: none.

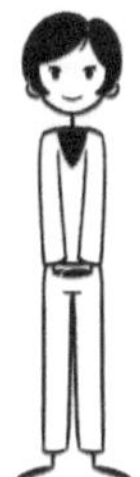 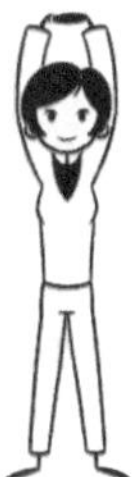

Ardha Sthambasana (partial position of the pillar)

Starting position: on the back, legs together and extended, arms stretched along the sides. Inhale slowly and deeply.

Asana: exhale slowly, lift a stretched leg to form a right angle with the torso.

Hold the position for five breaths, then inhale and exhale slowly bringing the legs back to the ground.

In the same way, repeat the execution of the asana with the other leg.

Benefits for the back: invigorates the back.

Other benefits: invigorates the pelvis and the muscles of the legs.

Contraindications: none.

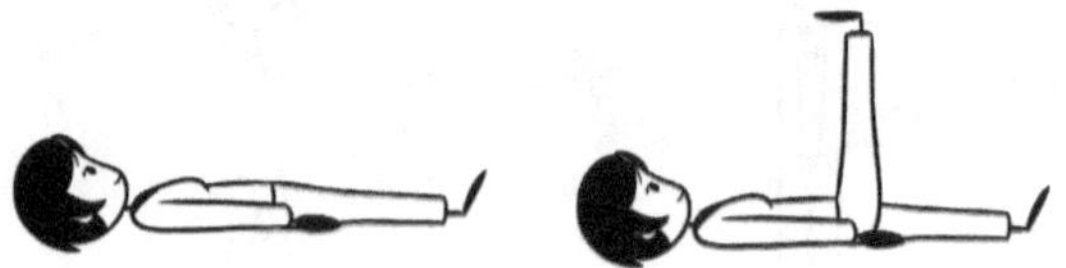

Bhujangasana (cobra pose)

Starting position: prone, legs and feet together, hands under the shoulders and facing the ground.

Asana: inhale deeply and slowly raise the head, slightly arching back the neck, shoulders and torso.

Exhale deeply and hold the position for 10 breaths, gradually increasing up to 20 with practice.

Then, breathing in and out, return to the starting position.

Benefits for the back: corrects the wrong positions of the spine toning the vertebrae, strengthens the back muscles.

Other benefits: strengthens the nervous system, keeps the kidneys healthy, facilitates digestion and maintains healthy the genital system.

Contraindications: do not perform the asana if you suffer from inguinal or dorsal hernia, or in weak or compromised abdominal organs.

In the case of cervical arthritis, start the asana by bringing the chin to the ground instead of the forehead and not arching the neck backwards.

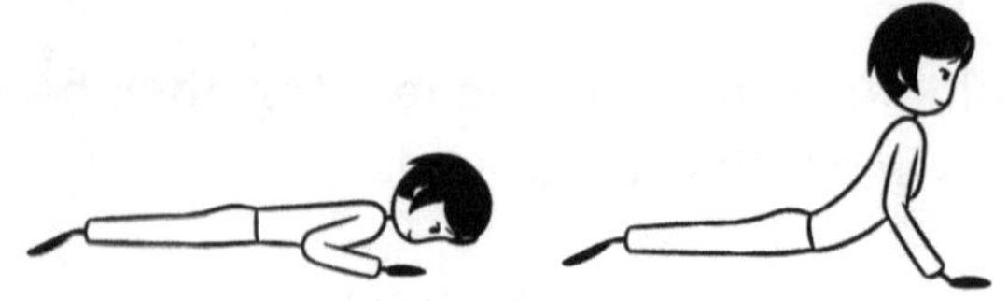

Chatushkonasana (position of the square)

Starting position: standing, straight back, legs straight, feet together and arms at the sides.

Asana: Inhale deeply, then exhale and flex the torso forward until it is parallel to the ground.

Push the shoulders back so as to keep the back straight, keeping the arms relaxed.

Hold the position during 10 breaths, then inhale slowly, lift up the torso and, returning to the starting position, exhale deeply.

Benefits for the back: tones the muscles of the back, strengthens the vertebral column.

Other benefits: tones the muscles of the abdomen.

Contraindications: none.

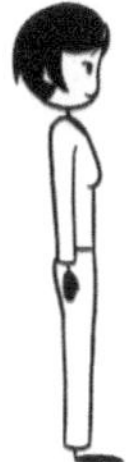 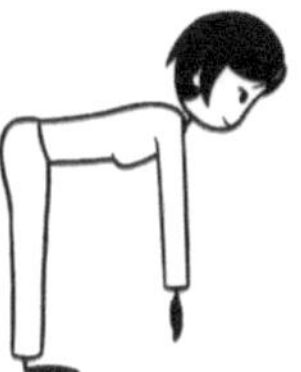

Dandasana (stick pose)

Starting position: on the back, with the arms along the body, legs and feet together.

Asana: breathing slowly and deeply, bring the arms outstretched beyond the head, hold the breath for a couple of seconds, stretch all the muscles, then make a slow and deep exhalation.

Hold the position for 10-20 breaths, to be performed normally.

Benefits for the back: corrects small deformations of the shoulders, eliminates back pain.

Other benefits: improves the functionality of the respiratory system, strengthens all the muscles (especially the abdominal muscles).

Contraindications: none.

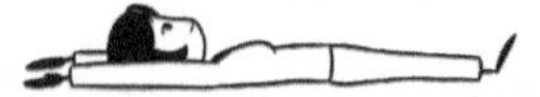

Dhanurasana (bow pose)

Starting position: prone, legs stretched, arms at the sides. Inhale and, while exhaling, slightly open the legs.

Breathe again and bend your legs.

Asana: exhaling, grasping the ankles, then, breathing in, arching back the neck and torso, raising the knees from the floor. Stretch out the whole body and exhale.

Hold the position initially for some breathing, gradually reaching up to 20 breaths with practice.

Inhale and, exhaling deeply, slowly return to the starting position (prone).

Benefits for the back: elasticizes the spine.

Other benefits: decongests the solar plexus by acting on the digestive system, tones the abdominal organs, keeps the kidneys healthy, helps in case of menstrual delays, eliminates the superfluous fat in the central part of the body, prevents and cures cellulite, increases respiratory capacity.

Contraindications: do not perform in case of liver and spleen, enlarged, weak abdominal organs, herniated discs or inguinal, cervical arthrosis.

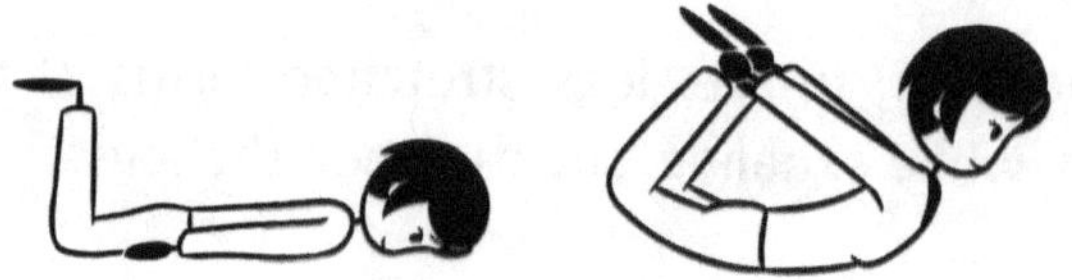

Dharmikasana (devotional pose)

Starting position: sitting on open heels, joined toes. Stretch the spine, inhale, and relax the shoulders, exhaling. After a couple of deep breaths, slowly flex the torso forward.

Asana: flexed bust, outstretched arms, forehead and nose to the ground, forearms adhering to the ground, hold position for 10-20 breaths.

Benefits for the back: relaxes the back and eliminates pain.

Other benefits: tones the internal abdominal organs, eliminates stomach ache and headaches.

Contraindications: in case of low blood pressure or cervical arthrosis, replace this position with Sadhasana. Women must avoid this position during menstruation, as this position tends to increase menstrual flow.

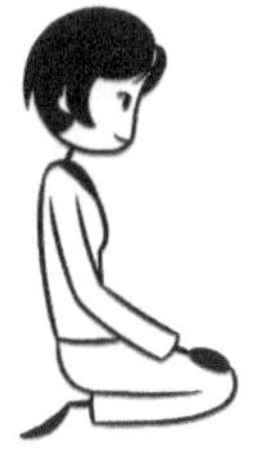 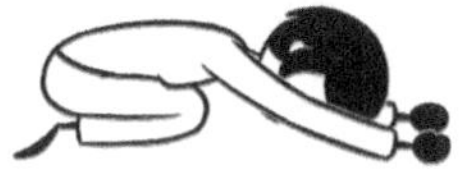

Ganapatiasana (Ganesha pose)

Starting position: standing, upright torso, legs and feet together, arms folded behind the back.

Inhale slowly and deeply. Exhale, flex the torso forward to be parallel to the floor.

Asana: raise a leg, taut, so that it is parallel to the ground. Maintain the position during 5-10 breaths.

Breathing in, lift the torso slowly, bringing the leg together again. Then repeat the asana on the other side.

Benefits for the back: tones the back.

Other benefits: improves the sense of balance and tones the legs.

Contraindications: none.

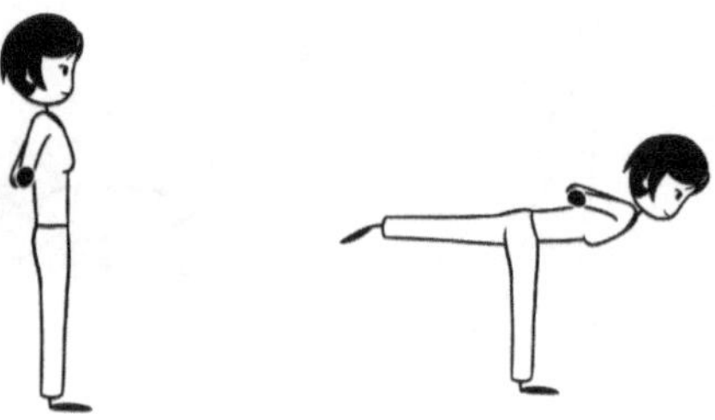

Gomukhasana (cow face pose)

Starting position: sitting on the ground, legs stretched out and apart, hands on the ground near the hips.

Cross the legs on each other, bending them. Bring your arms out.

Asana: flex the arms behind the back, one from the top and the other from the bottom. Grasp your hands and hold the position during 5-10 breaths.

Finally return with the arms out and repeat the execution of the asana on the other side.

Benefits for the back: straightens the back, elasticizes the shoulder joint.

Other benefits: develops the chest, improving breathing, facilitates digestion, purifies the bronchi, curates and prevents facial acne.

Contraindications: none.

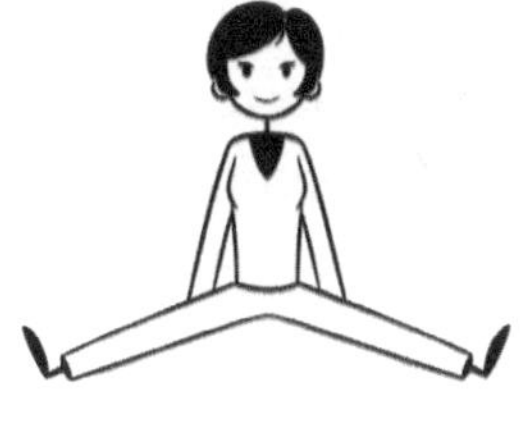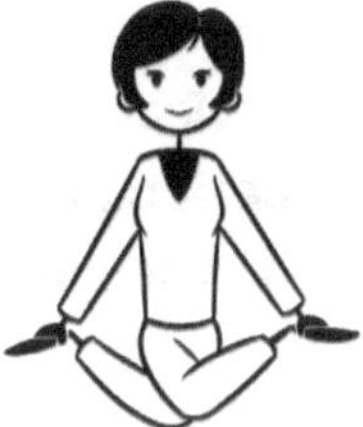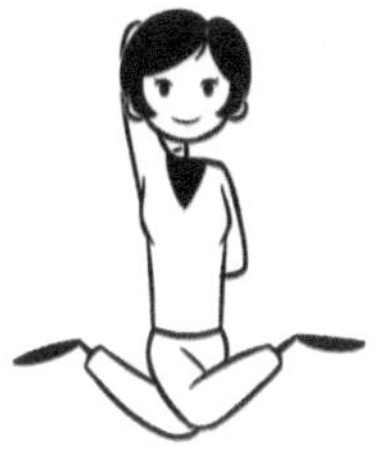

Halasana (plow pose)

Starting position: supine, legs stretched, feet together, arms at the sides. Inhale and raise the legs together and stretched, until forming a right angle with the pelvis. Exhale.

Asana: breathing in, lift the pelvis off the floor and bring the legs outstretched beyond the head until it touches the ground with the toes. Exhale and maintain position for 5-10 breaths.

Inhaling, lift your feet off the ground and exhaling return with your back to the ground, forming a right angle again between your legs and pelvis.

Exhale and return with your legs on the ground in the starting position.

Benefits for the back: elasticizes the spine.

Other benefits: stimulates the endocrine glands, massages the abdominal organs, stimulates and drains liver and pancreas, useful for those suffering from diabetes, regularizes the functioning of the thyroid, lowers the blood pressure if the asana is maintained for 10- 15 minutes.

Contraindications: disc hernias, deviation of the vertebral column, hyperthyroidism, cervical arthrosis. Avoid performing the asana in the menstrual period and in case of inflammation of the throat or face. Suspend the execution if there is sudden heat to the head.

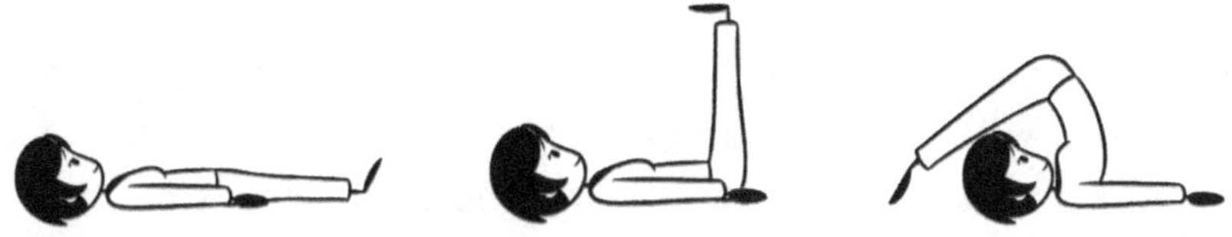

Jathara Parivartanasana (revolved abdomen pose)

Starting position: supine, open arms, palms facing up, legs together. With an inhalation, flex your legs with your knees together. With an exhalation bring the legs, always holding them together and bent, on one side.

Asana: the legs should rest on the ground, adherent and relaxed. Hold the position for 5-10 breaths, then inhale, lift the legs together again and, expiring, spread them on the ground in the starting position.

Repeat the asana on the other side in the same way.

Benefits for the back: eliminates back pain.

Other benefits: invigorates the liver, spleen and pancreas, strengthens the intestine, treats gastritis, elasticizes the hips and reduces fat.

Contraindications: none.

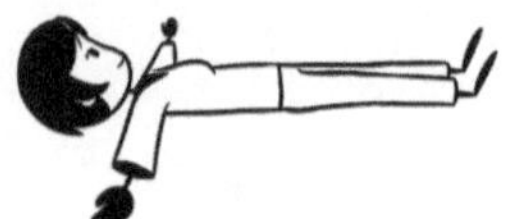 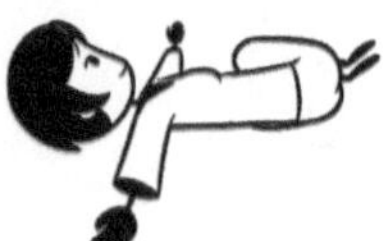 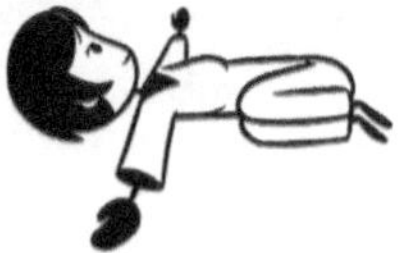

Matsyasana (fish pose)

Starting position: seated, legs together and stretched forward, hands on hips. Inhale deeply and, exhaling, bend the torso backwards, bringing the forearms to the ground.

Asana: breathing deeply, push the chest out and, exhaling, slide the arms forward and backwards, until touching the ground with the nape of the neck.

The hands are resting on the thighs, the elbows on the ground as well as the pelvis. Hold the position for 5-10 breaths, to be gradually increased.

Inhaling and exhaling, let yourself finally slip to the ground.

Benefits for the back: tones the lumbo-sacral region.

Other benefits: it is effective against constipation, chronic bronchitis, asthma, prevents reflexes and inflammation of the throat, tones the genital apparatus and the nervous system.

Contraindications: do not perform if you suffer from cervical arthritis.

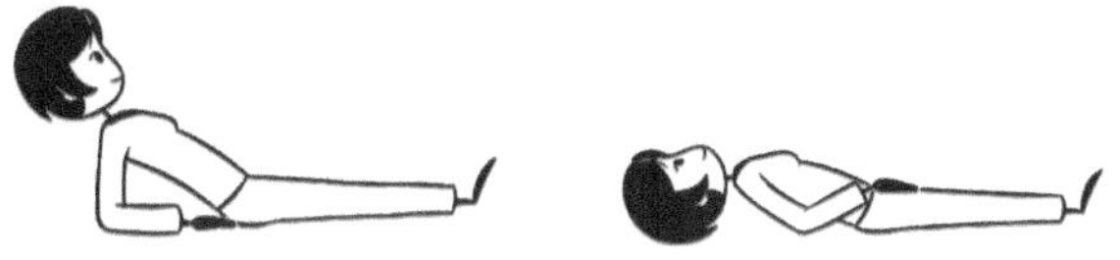

Natarajasana (lord of the dance pose)

Starting position: standing, inhale raising one arm at the top and at the same time flexing the other leg backwards.

Asana: grasping the instep of the corresponding raised leg with your hand (for example the right hand, grab the right foot). Exhale slowly, flex the torso forward.

Hold the position for 10-15 breaths, then inhale, bring your upper body upright and, exhaling, lower your arms and legs.

Benefits for the back: strengthens the muscles of the torso, elasticizes the spine.

Other benefits: strengthens the muscles of the legs and arms, improves the sense of balance and facilitates digestion.

Contraindications: none.

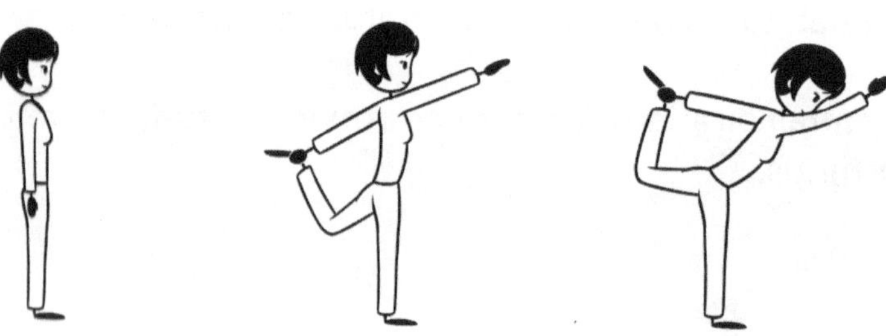

Pakshi asana (stork bird pose)

Starting position: standing, legs stretched, feet together. Inhale slowly.

Asana: exhaling, flexing the torso forward, turning back the shoulders and slightly arching the back.

At the same time, lift the outstretched arms back, with the palms facing up and maintain the position for 5-10 breaths, focusing on the spine.

Inhale, lift the torso slowly and, exhaling, return to the starting position.

Benefits for the back: invigorates the muscles of the back, strengthens the spine and straightens the rounded shoulders.

Other benefits: invigorates the muscles of the abdomen and legs.

Contraindications: none.

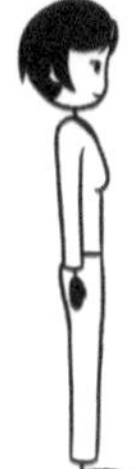 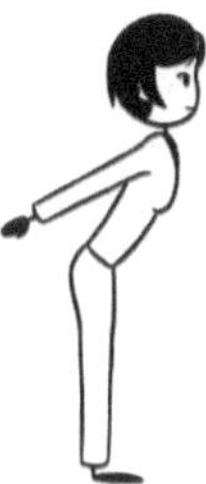

Paripurna Navasana (rowing boat pose)

Starting position: sitting on the ground, legs extended forward and united, hands on the sides of the thighs. Inhaling, bring your hands to the ground.

Asana: exhale, lift the legs (holding them together), bring the weight of the body back, pivoting on the sacral area, and remove the hands from the ground bringing them, with the arms outstretched, to the sides of the knees. Hold this position for 3-4 breaths, gradually increasing up to 10 with training.

Benefits for the back: strengthens the lumbosacral area.

Other benefits: massages the abdominal muscles, deflates the abdomen from the gas, slims the abdominal area.

Contraindications: avoid if you suffer from enlarged liver.

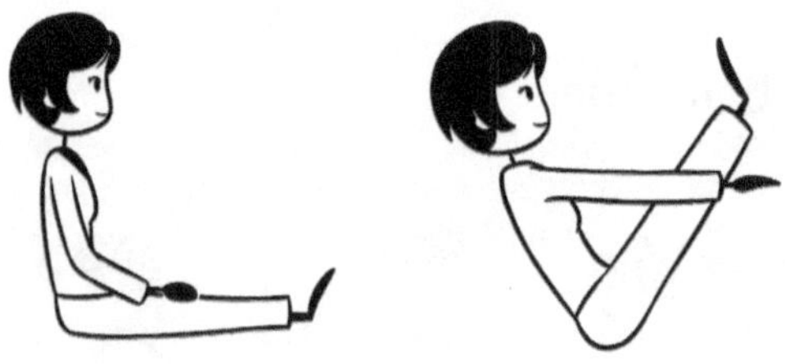

Parivrtta Trikonasana (revolved triangle pose)

Starting position: standing, legs apart, arms at the sides. Inhaling, bring your arms out to shoulder height.

Asana: exhale, bend the torso to one side and pull the opposite ankle with your hand (for example, right hand on left ankle).

Keeping the legs outstretched, the other arm rises upwards with the palm of the hand pointing outwards.

Focus on the spine that stretches with each breath and maintain the asana during 5-20 breaths.

Inhaling, slowly raise the torso, bringing the arms parallel to the ground. Exhale, lower the arms. Repeat the asana on the other side.

Benefits for the back: invigorates the back muscles, elasticizes the spine.

Other benefits: invigorates the abdominal organs, strengthens the legs.

Contraindications: none.

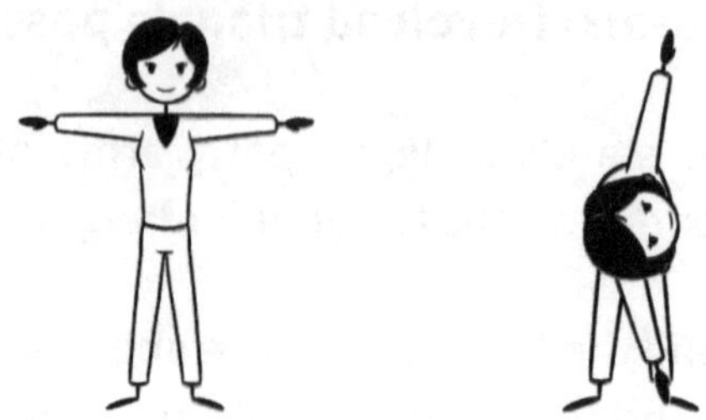

Parsvottanasana (pyramid pose)

Starting position: standing, upright torso, legs stretched out and feet together. Hands are clasped behind the back, fingers pointing up.

Inhale. Exhale, turn the torso to one side at the same time as the corresponding leg, so that the feet form a right angle.

Inhaling, slightly arching back the back and, expiring, flex the trunk forward so that it is parallel to the ground.

Asana: inhale and, by exhaling, fully flex the torso, bringing the forehead to the knee.

Stay in this position during 5 breaths, gradually increasing with practice up to 20.

To return to the starting position, inhale and slowly raise the face first and then the upper body. Exhale, turn the torso back to its initial position. Inhale, join your feet and relax your arms.

Repeat the asana on the other side in the same way.

Benefits for the back: tones the muscles of the back, straightens the shoulders.

Other benefits: massages the abdominal organs, facilitates digestion, tones the muscles of the legs and arms.

Contraindications: if you suffer from high or low pressure, finish the asana without returning to the starting position.

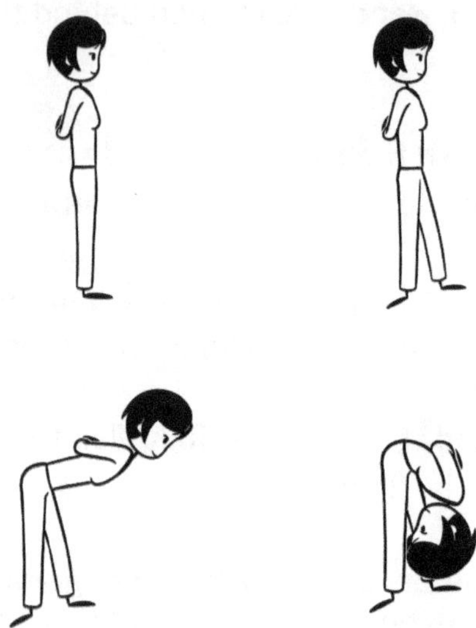

Parsvottanasana (pyramid pose) - variation

Starting position: standing, legs apart and slightly divergent feet. Inhale deeply and flex the torso forward, rotating it slightly to one side.

Asana: grasp the ankle with both hands, resting the forehead on the knee. Hold the position for 5-10 breaths.

Inhale, slowly raise your torso and turn it forward. Repeat the asana with the other leg.

Benefits for the back: elasticizes the spine.

Other benefits: elasticizes the legs and hips. If the asana is performed during the menstrual period, it reduces the flow.

Contraindications: if you suffer from low blood pressure, instead of resting your forehead on your knee, stay with your torso parallel to the ground, with your arms outstretched and looking upwards.

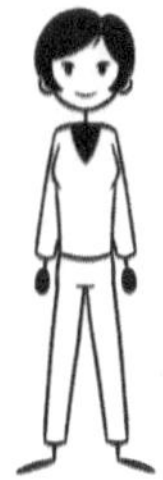
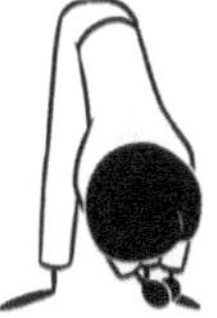

Purvottanasana (upward plank pose)

Starting position: sitting on the ground, legs extended forward and united, arms extended with hands resting on the ground on the sides of the buttocks.

Asana: breathing in, raising the pelvis and, breathing out, arching the body backwards lengthening it. Hold the position for 3-4 breaths, then return to the sitting position by inhaling and exhaling slowly.

Benefits for the back: elasticizes the spine, tones and strengthens the dorsal muscles, corrects incorrect back postures.

Other benefits: tones and strengthens the abdominal muscles.

Contraindications: do not perform if you suffer from inguinal hernias or discs.

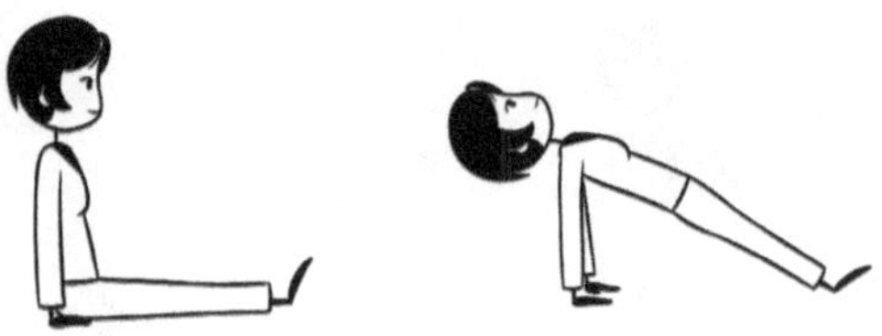

Sadhakasana (pose of the adept)

Starting position: sitting on heels, joined toes.

Asana: slowly flex the torso forward and at the same time close the fists with the thumbs inside. Bring your forearms to the ground with your elbows close to your knees and rest your forehead against the overlapping fists.

In performing this posture, perform a couple of breaths in the starting position, lengthening the spine in the inspiratory phase and relaxing the shoulders in the exhalation phase. Then take the asana (with the inflected bust) for ten breaths.

Benefits for the back: relaxes the back and eliminates pain.

Other benefits: tones the internal organs of the abdomen, is effective against stomach ache and headaches.

Contraindications: none.

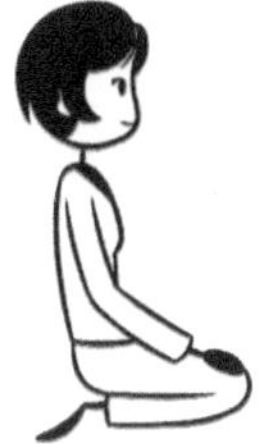
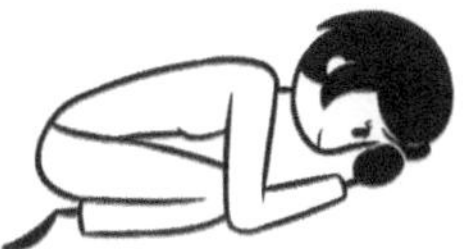

Sayana Buddhasana (reclining Buddha pose)

Starting position: in this particular asana, the starting position and the asana coincide. Lying on one side, with one arm resting on the ground, the folded forearm and one hand supporting the head (keep the wrist at the temple, the palm of the hand resting on the ear and the fingers on the neck). The other arm is distended on the side.

Resume the whole body and hold the position for 10-20 breaths on each side.

Benefits: relaxes body and mind.

Contraindications: none.

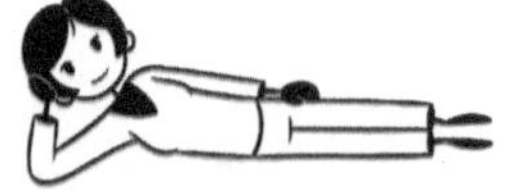

Setu Bandhasana (bridge pose)

Starting position: lying down with legs apart and bent, hands gripping the ankles, feet resting on the ground with the soles of the feet well adherent to the floor.

Asana: inhale deeply and lift the pelvis, maintaining the position for five breaths, trying to push the abdomen upward with each breath.

Gradually the number of breaths can be increased up to 20.

Benefits for the back: strengthens the spine.

Other benefits: tones all the muscles, increases the chest volume and improves normal breathing.

Contraindications: none.

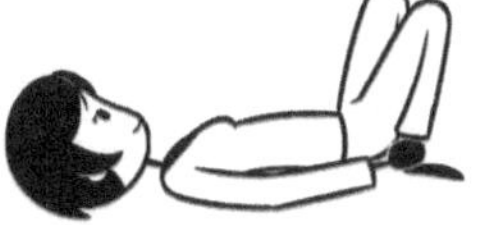 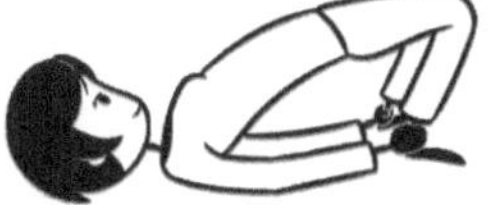

Sthambasana (pillar pose)

Starting position: on the back, legs together, arms stretched along the sides. Inhale deeply.

Asana: exhaling, raising arms and legs so as to form two right angles with the torso. With your back firmly on the ground, hold the position for 5-10 breaths.

Finish the asana by inhaling deeply and, exhaling slowly, bring your arms and legs back to the ground.

Benefits for the back: invigorates the muscles of the back.

Other benefits: invigorates the pelvis and the muscles of the legs.

Contraindications: none.

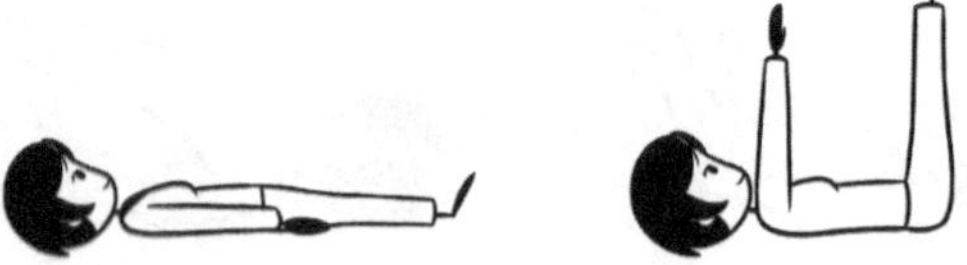

Sukhasana (easy pose)

Seated, legs crossed. Keep your torso upright, with the shoulders stretched backwards, arms relaxed, hands on knees. Relax your feet and legs, arms, neck and face. By maintaining this posture, all respiratory exercises can be performed.

Benefits for the back: strengthens the back.

Other benefits: tones the pelvis.

Contraindications: none.

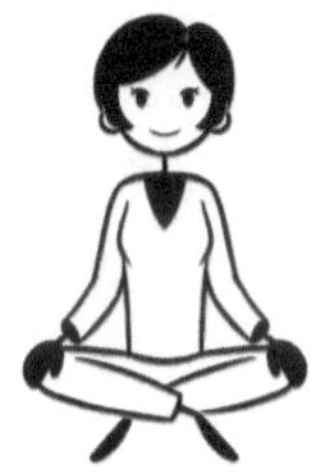

Supta Konasana (reclining bound angle pose)

Starting position: on the back, bend the legs and spread them apart. Inhaling, join the feet and grasp the two toes with your hands.

Asana: exhaling, stretching the legs and arms, making the back adhere perfectly to the ground. Hold the position for 5-10 breaths.

Benefits for the back: strengthens the back.

Other benefits: useful for the blood circulation of the legs and pelvis, elasticizes the perineum.

Contraindications: none.

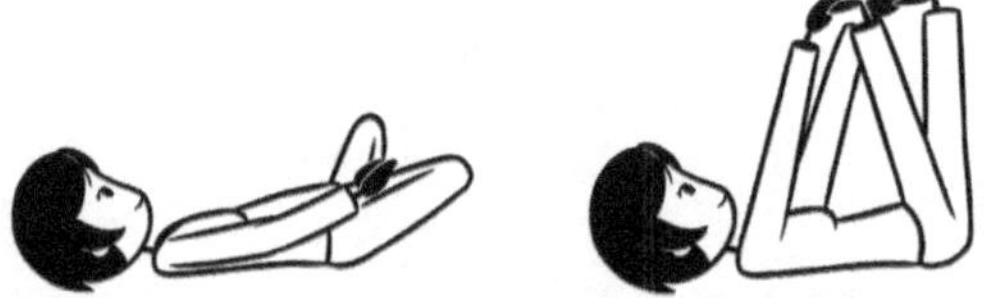

Surya Namaskara (sun salutation)

The "greeting to the sun" connects a series of twelve asanas to be performed in sequence and is perfect for both starting and ending a yoga session.

Pranamasana (prayer pose): standing with legs outstretched and feet together, join hands on chest in prayer position.

Hasta Uttanasana (raised arms pose): perform two or three deep breaths, then inhale deeply and raise the upper arms, arching the torso backwards.

Hasta Padasana (hand-to-foot pose): exhale, bend the torso forward and bring your hands on the ground.

Ashwa Sanchalanasana (equestrian pose): inhale, stretch back one leg, resting on the ground the knee and the back of the foot, bending the other.

Parvatasana (mountain pose): hold the breath for a second, put the feet backwards, pointing them to the ground, and spread the legs bringing up the pelvis and forming a bridge.

Chaturanga Dandasana (four-limbed staff pose): exhale deeply and let the body slide to the floor.

Bhujangasana (cobra pose): breathing in, stretch out your arms by lifting your torso. The gaze is turned upwards.

Parvatasana (mountain pose): exhale, return to the mountain position again, with the legs and arms outstretched and the pelvis at the top.

Ashwa Sanchalanasana (equestrian pose): inhaling, carrying forward the foot that had previously been left behind. Bend the leg and stretch back the other knee and the back of the foot that adhere to the ground.

Hasta Padasana (hand-to-foot pose): exhaling, bringing together the feet, legs stretched out. With the torso bent forward bring your hands to the ankles.

Hasta Uttanasana (raised arms pose): inhale, lift the torso, arching it backwards and lift the arms upwards.

Pranamasana (prayer pose): breathing out, rejoining the hands on the chest in prayer position, returning to the starting position.

Benefits for the back: elasticizes the vertebral column.

Other benefits: tones all the abdominal organs, improving digestion and intestinal transit; strengthens the muscles of the whole body, improves respiratory capacity.

Executed in the morning, as soon as you get up, it prepares your body and mind to face the day.

Performed in the evening, before going to bed, it combines sleep.

Contraindications: none.

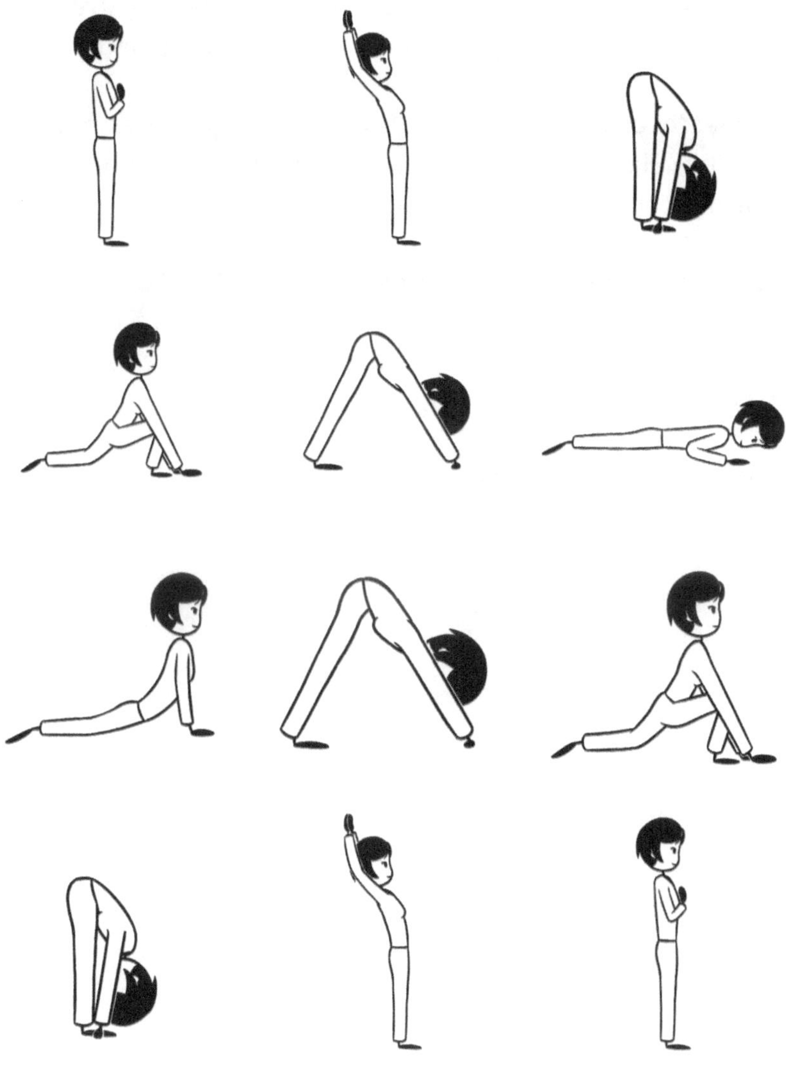

Tadasana (mountain pose)

Starting position: standing, upright torso, legs outstretched, feet together, arms slightly open, hands outstretched.

Asana: focus on the spine and try to straighten it as much as possible. Hold the position for a few minutes while remaining still and concentrate on breathing.

Benefits for the back: strengthens the back.

Other benefits: strengthens the legs, increases physical and mental strength, memory and concentration.

Contraindications: none.

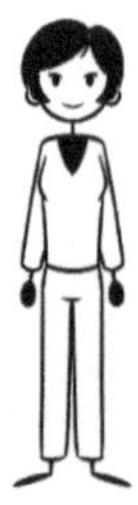

Trikonasana (triangle pose)

Starting position: standing, legs apart, arms out at shoulder height.

Inhaling, turn one foot outwards.

Asana: exhale, slowly flex the torso from the part of the foot you have just turned outward and take the calf or, if possible, the ankle with your hand.

Keep the other arm stretched up, legs outstretched, and look up at the raised hand. Stay in this position for 5-10 breaths, then inhale slowly, lift your upper body and bring your arms out to shoulder height.

Rotate the foot and bring it back to its original position. Repeat the asana on the other side.

Benefits for the back: tones the muscles of the back.

Other benefits: develops the chest improving breathing, tones the muscles of the legs, elasticizes the hips and ankles and corrects the malformations of the legs.

Contraindications: none.

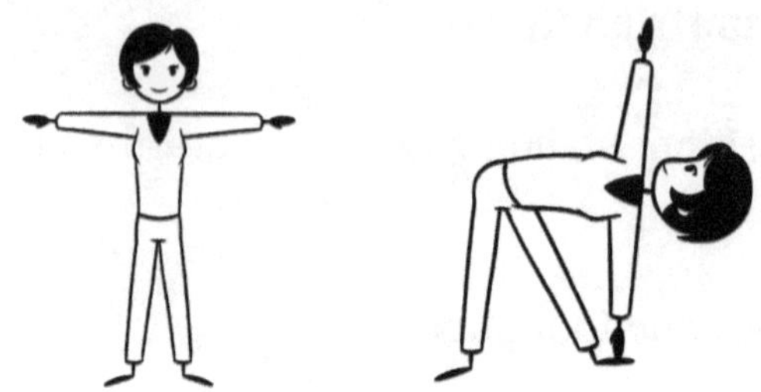

Ugrasana (ferocious pose)

Starting position: sitting on the ground, upright torso, legs stretched together and torso and legs form a right angle. Hands are on the knees.

Inhale, stretch the spine lengthening the torso; exhale, relax your shoulders.

Repeat several times before starting the asana.

Asana: inhale deeply and, exhaling, bend the torso forward by grasping the feet or ankles. The elbows must touch the ground.

Hold the position for some breathing and then gradually increase to keep it for a few minutes.

Inhale slowly in raising the upper body.

Benefits for the back: tones the vertebral column.

Other benefits: massage the whole genital apparatus, keeping it healthy; tones the abdomen, the kidneys and the nervous system; improves diuresis, eliminates headaches.

Contraindications: avoid practicing this asana during menstruation.

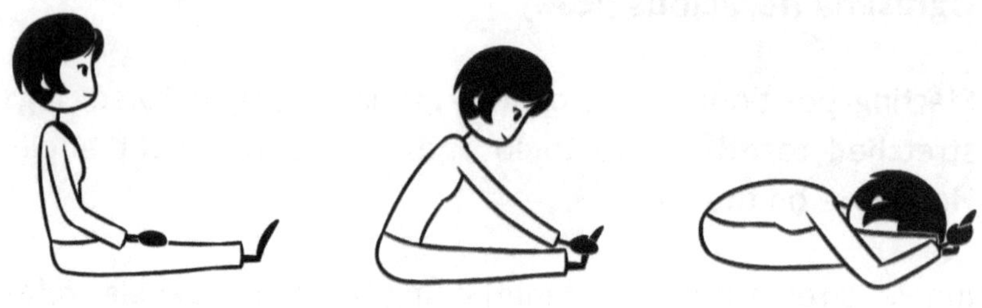

70

Ustrasana (camel pose)

Starting position: kneeling, hands on hips with thumbs touching behind the back, legs and thighs forming a right angle.

Inhale deeply and push the chest out. Exhale, bring back gradually (in this order) the head, shoulders and torso, pushing out chest and abdomen.

Asana: stretch out your arms until you catch the heels. Push the abdomen out, inhaling, so as to make arms and legs parallel.

Hold the position for some breathing then, inhaling, slowly raise the torso and exhale to sit back on the heels again.

With practice get to hold the position for 10-20 breaths.

Benefits for the back: tones the entire spine, straightens the shoulders.

Other benefits: tones the genital and urinary system, keeps the kidneys healthy, increases diuresis, strengthens the abdomen and pelvis, facilitates the elimination of toxins, eliminates unnecessary fat from the abdomen and hips.

Contraindications: hyperthyroidism, enlarged liver or spleen, weak or compromised abdominal organs, inguinal hernia or slipped disc.

Stop performing the asana if you feel a sudden heat in your face, a whistling in your ears, a burning sensation in your eyes or a strong tension in the kidney area.

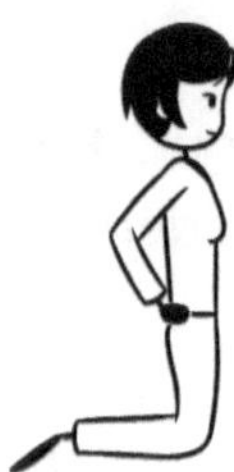 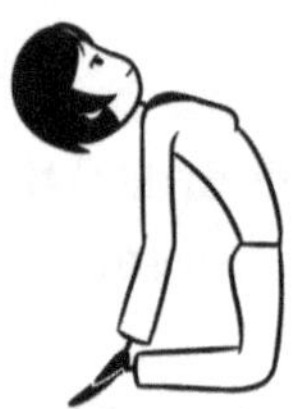

Utkatasana (chair pose)

Starting position: standing, straight back, legs stretched out, knees and feet together, palms of hands together forward.

Asana: breathing slowly and deeply, bring your arms above your head, keeping your hands together. Exhale, bend the legs trying to keep the soles of the feet close to the ground.

Hold the position for 10-20 breaths, without lifting the heels off the ground and keeping the knee joint.

Finally inhale, stretch out the legs. Exhale and bring your arms back down.

Benefits for the back: tones the back, elasticize shoulders and ankles.

Other benefits: gently massage the heart, increase the breathing capacity, tones the abdomen, corrects the malformations of the legs and feet.

Contraindications: none.

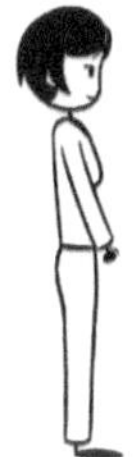
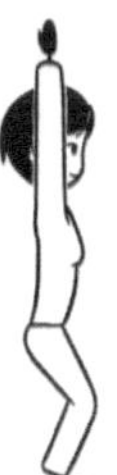

Uttanasa (standing forward bend pose)

Starting position: standing, legs slightly apart. Inhale deeply. Exhale deeply and lean the torso slowly forward, so you can grasp the ankles with your hands.

Keep your legs stretched and look forward.

Asana: inhale and exhale bend the elbows, flexing the torso until the head is between the legs.

Hold the position 5-10 breaths, then inhale, raise the head very slowly and then the upper body. Exhale.

Benefits for the back: elasticizes the vertebral column.

Other benefits: stimulates the pituitary, tones the abdominal organs, corrects small deformations in the legs.

Contraindications: none.

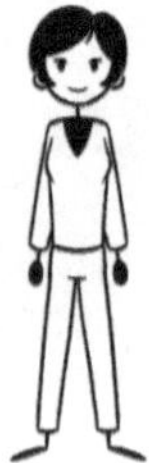 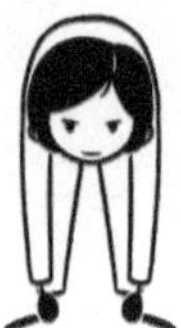 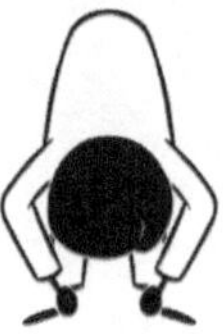

Utthita Konasana (extended side angle pose)

Starting position: sitting on the ground, legs extended forward and united. After a deep inhalation, flex the torso forward by exhaling and grasping a foot with the corresponding hand, pressing on the knee of the same leg with the other hand.

Asana: breathing in, raising the leg while maintaining elongation. Stay in this position for a duration of 5-10 breaths. Repeat with the same procedures on the other leg.

Benefits for the back: strengthens and tones the muscles of the back.

Other benefits: strengthens and tones the muscles of the legs.

Contraindications: none.

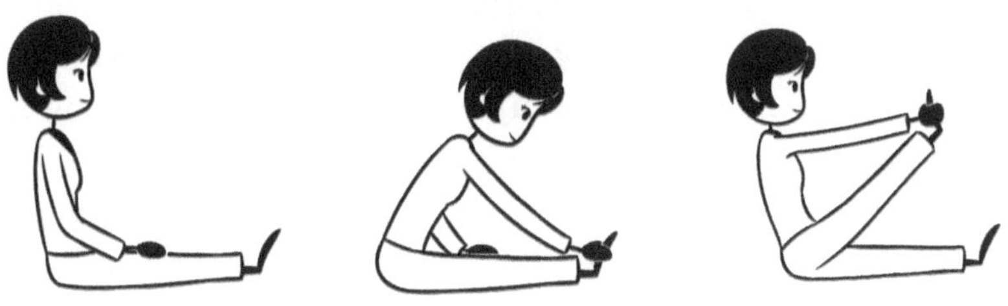

Pranayama

In this chapter we will talk about the techniques of pranayama. What they are, how they should be performed and what benefits they bring to our psycho-physical health.

We will also describe in detail three pranayama exercises that we will use in the series of exercises that you will find at the end of the book, which combine yoga asanas, with pranayama techniques and relaxation exercises, with the aim of eliminating back pain.

What are pranayamas?

The word pranayama (in Sanskrit प्राणायाम) can be translated as "breath control" and is composed from the words in Sanskrit "prana" (vital energy or breath) and "ayama" (control, length, expansion, in relation to breathing).

According to Hindu physiology, all living beings, are endowed with prana, whose conservation derives from the correct development of all the psychological, emotional and physiological functions necessary for the harmonious maintenance of the inner equilibrium.

One of the forms through which prana can be obtained (in fact, we can say that it is the main form) is precisely through the breathing, which brings into our body in addition to oxygen, also the vital energy (understood as subtle energy) present in the air.

The concept of prana (understood as vital breath or energy) is fundamental in Indian culture and, more generally, in yoga. Here we will mention only a few basic concepts, which will help to better understand the importance of pranayama.

Prana consists of five distinct energetic currents (or vayus, translatable as "air"), each of which performs a distinct action and presides certain vital functions in the different areas of the body.

Prana: refers to the inspiratory phase, to the air that is inhaled, drawing the life force.

Apana: responsible for the expiratory phase. Apana regulates the functions of the digestive system, ejaculation and childbirth in women.

Udana: it is the energy (or air) that rises from the throat and is responsible for regulating lung function and swallowing. It also instructs to raise the energy of kundalini.

Samana: it is the energy that crosses the central part of the body. It is associated with the functions of thermoregulation, digestion and the circulation of nutrients in the body.

Vyana: it is the energy that circulates and spreads throughout the body, responsible for metabolism and blood circulation.

The breathing control techniques (pranayama) are therefore an indispensable tool for getting to know your body, as well as for achieving that balance between body and mind which is the basis for maintaining good health.

How to practice pranayamas

Unlike other involuntary processes that occur in our body, such as digestion, breathing is an involuntary act on which we can partially intervene. For example, we can decide to take deep breaths or hold our breath for a longer or shorter period depending on the capacity of each person.

This happens because respiratory activity is an involuntary process regulated by nerve centers which, in turn, can be partially inhibited by other cerebral impulses at a more conscious level, which allows us to decide "how" we want to breathe.

We can distinguish three different types of breathing, each of which acts on a distinct parts of the body, performing a distinct action on a physiological level.

The first is abdominal breathing, which mainly uses the lower part of the lungs. During inhalation, thanks to the function exerted by the diaphragm, the abdomen swells and creates a depression in the rib cage that causes the lungs to dilate and the air to penetrate deeply. In the expiration phase the diaphragm rises and creates an increase in pressure in the rib cage which causes the lungs to be emptied and the abdomen to be deflated.

Deep abdominal breathing is the one that allows the greatest exchange of air. This type of breathing allows in fact obtaining a good oxygenation of the arterial blood and creates a healthy pressure on the internal organs, making a continuous massage.

During thoracic respiration, on the other hand, the central and upper part of the lungs is mainly used. During the inhalation phase the thoracic cavity is dilated and the lungs are expanded, allowing the air to penetrate. During expiration, the intercostal muscles contract by decreasing the thoracic volume and pushing the air out of the chest. The amount of air that enters is less than that of abdominal breathing.

Finally, the upper part of the lungs is mainly used in clavicular respiration. Air enters the lungs by moving the clavicles and shoulders upward. The amount of air that enters the lungs is minimal compared to the previous types of breathing.

When these three types of breathing are performed simultaneously, without interruption between one cycle and the other, we are performing a complete yogic breathing, which allows the lungs to function at their maximum capacity.

During a normal yoga session usually pranayama exercises are performed in a simple meditative position, such as Sukhasana. However, this is not a necessary requirement, also because many people may have difficulty, especially at the beginning, in maintaining such a position even for short periods of time, since they would feel joint pains.

The good news is that anyone, at any age, can practice pranayama techniques, because the meditative position can be replaced by any other position in which, basically, one feels comfortable and relaxed.

For example, you can sit cross-legged, using cushions under your knees or your butt, or even sitting on a chair, with your soles resting on the ground. The important thing is to maintain a comfortable, stable, relaxed posture and keep the back straight, with the head aligned to the vertebral column.

It is especially important to try to relax the muscles of the body during the practice of pranayama, since this state of physical relaxation also helps to dissolve mental tensions, with consequent benefit on physiological functions.

General benefits of pranayamas

The regular practice of pranayama exercises produces a series of overall benefits on the body and mind, due to the fact that their main function is to increase the intake of oxygen in the blood and eliminate the excesses of carbon dioxide, taking enormous benefits from cells and tissues of the body.

The mental and physical benefits of pranayama are numerous. Within the most important are:

- facilitates the elimination of toxins

- improves blood and lymphatic circulation

- optimizes the filtering action of the kidneys

- tones the nervous system

- acts positively on the memory

- helps digestion

- stimulates the spleen

- balances the glandular system

- strengthens the immune system

- increases lung capacity

- generates peace of mind

- helps reduce stress and anxiety

- helps to sleep well

List of breathing exercises (Pranayamas)

Below you will find a list of three pranayamas, which used in combination with previously described yoga asanas, help to restore the psycho-physical balance necessary to regain back health and eliminate pain.

Ujjayi Pranayama (respiration of the victorious)

You can perform this breathing technique while sitting, lying on the back or even walking.

Inhale and exhale normally, trying to relax the shoulders, neck, jaw and muscles of the face.

Inhale again with the nose and exhale with it from the mouth, emitting a light sound similar to what we would do by trying to tarnish a glass or whispering.

Try to repeat the same sound during the inhalation with the nose and, when you feel comfortable, realize the entire inhalation and exhalation cycle only through the nose.

Start by taking 10 breaths a day, gradually increasing up to 5 minutes of practice.

Thanks to this breathing technique you can consciously restrict the opening of the glottis (normally controlled in an unconscious manner), so that the air stays longer in the pharynx and nasal cavities.

It is important, especially when you start practicing this pranayama, to remember that the breath must be slow, deep and above all regular, trying not to over-close the glottis (otherwise you risk not blocking excessively the air flow).

Benefits:

• slows the heartbeat

• improves the functioning of the circulatory system

• produces a warming effect in the body, increasing body temperature

• calms your mind

• increases the elasticity of the lungs

• relieves stress and reduces nervous tension

• helps to fight insomnia

Complete yogic breathing

Seated, back straight and eyes half shut.

In order to perform complete yogic breathing correctly, it will be necessary to divide the breathing into three distinct phases: abdominal, thoracic and clavicular.

Only when breathing will be learned in its three different phases will it be possible to switch to full yogic breathing, where the abdomen will swell in one deep inhalation, the ribcage will open and the clavicles will rise slightly.

Similarly, during the expiration phase, the abdomen will deflate, the ribcage will close and the clavicles will be lowered.

Let's see, separately, the three phases of complete yogic respiration.

Abdominal breathing: place your hands on the abdomen, without compressing it. Inhale slowly and deeply, slightly inflating the abdomen. Exhale, deflate it. Repeat for some respiratory acts.

Chest breathing: place your hands on the ribcage. Inhale slowly and deeply, open the ribcage. Exhale, close it. Repeat for some respiratory acts.

Clavicular breathing: place hands at the base of the neck. Inhale slowly and deeply, lift the clavicles. Exhale, lower them. Repeat for some respiratory acts.

Once breathing has been learned in its three phases, complete yogic breathing can be practiced in cycles of 5 or 10 inspirations and expirations.

Benefits:

- maintains the health of the lungs

- calms the mind and body

- reduces stress and anxiety

- reduces muscle tension

- increases the supply of oxygen in the blood

Surya – Chandra Pranayama (single nostril breathing)

This breathing exercise combines two types of pranayama: Surya Bheda, or Sun piercing breath, and Chandra Bheda, or Moon piercing breath.

In the solar breathing technique, only the right nostril is used, while in the lunar one the left nostril is used. This pranayama instead is performed by alternating the nostrils.

Sitting comfortably with the back straight, close the left nostril with the ring finger and the little finger of the right hand and inhale slowly and deeply from the right nostril. Hold the breath for 5 seconds, then close the right nostril with the thumb of the right hand and exhale deeply from the left nostril.

Close the left nostril again as explained above and repeat the breathing cycle for a few minutes.

Benefits:

• reduces stress and nervous tension

• revitalizes the body by improving circulation of *prana*

Mudras

In this chapter we will talk about mudras. What they are, how they should be performed and what benefits they bring to our psycho-physical health.

We will also describe in detail two body mudras that we will use in the series of exercises that you will find at the end of the book, which combine yoga asanas, with pranayama techniques and relaxation exercises, with the aim of eliminating back pain.

What are mudras?

It is defined as mudra (in Sanskrit मुद्रा, literally translatable as "seal" or "gesture"), a symbolic gesture that is used both in Hindu and Buddhist tradition, to obtain benefits on the physical, energetic and spiritual level.

Normally the mudras are usually performed with the hands, even if some mudras involve the whole body, in the form of gestures, movements or dances, or particular position of the eyes, and their use in the practice of yoga is usually associated with the completion of some asanas or during meditation, together with pranayama.

Mudras are part of a system that uses the body to express and emphasize the intentions of the mind for healing purposes, stimulating the flow of prana, or vital energy, of which all living beings are endowed. But, what does it means?

As mentioned also in the introduction of this book, we will not go into the details of the philosophical aspects that accompany yoga; nor will we go deeply into the theory that supports the effectiveness of the mudra and their healing power.

We will limit ourselves to mentioning that the symbolic positions assumed during the mudras represent some states of consciousness, which in turn manifest themselves on a physical or mental level, conveying a certain energetic quality or a particular type of vibration.

For example, the frequent and convicted realization of Agni Mudra (or gesture of fire) will result in an improvement of diseases related to digestion on the physical plane.

On the energetic level, according to yoga, the right hand represents the sun, while the left hand represents the moon. Furthermore, each finger of the hand represents a relationship between the elements and a distinct type of energy.

Briefly, the thumb corresponds to *Agni* (fire), to the index finger *Vayu* (air), to the middle finger *Akash* (space), to the ring finger *Prithvi* (earth) and to the little finger *Jar* (water).

In the classic yoga text *Gheranda Samhita* 25 fundamental mudra are listed, and another 108 are mentioned in Tantric texts, but in this book we will focus only on two of them, which have a special beneficial effect on back pain.

How to practice mudras

As we mentioned earlier, there are mudras that are made with the hands (most of them) and mudras that are performed with the body (those we will see in this book).

The execution of one or the other, however, has many aspects in common, since the mudra is basically a form of conveying energy through the body (or, better said, through the "seal" symbolized through the adopted posture).

In this sense, therefore, it makes no difference that we are doing a mudra with our hands or a mudra with our body. The main element in the practice of these exercises, and that basically is common to the whole practice of yoga, is the absence of tension.

It is important to perform the mudras in a state of relaxation, since any tension (both mental and physical) would prevent the flow of energy, which is instead the ultimate goal of the mudra.

The mudras we will see in this book are practiced from a sitting position. It will therefore be important to make sure that the posture we have adopted is symmetrical, with the back straight and the column aligned. It is therefore advisable to sit in a stable and comfortable way, and only once you have met the right position, begin the practice of mudra.

In the event that, for example, the knees do not comfortably rest on the ground or prevent us from maintaining a stable position, it is possible to help with cushions, so also (and above all) to ensure that the knees are at the same height and maintain the symmetry that we seek in practice (both vertical and horizontal).

Breathing also plays a very important role in the practice of body mudras. Just as the position must be stable and relaxed, the breathing must be smooth and fluid.

At the beginning it may be complicated to coordinate the gestures of the body and breathing, as well as rest in the yoga asanas, but soon you will realize how this connection is fundamental and will naturally turn out to accompany each gesture with the corresponding inhalation or exhalation.

We have talked about posture and breathing so far, the importance of avoiding physical and mental tensions and maintaining a regular rhythm of breathing.

However there is one last aspect to take into consideration, more mental than the previous ones; and it is that of awareness and visualization.

It is ideal to try to maintain a meditative attitude during the execution of the mudra, focusing on one's body, on physical sensations, on the observation of breathing, but also by practicing visualization, projecting mentally the image of the result we wish to obtain from the practice of mudra.

This last consideration must be bound to the fact that the mudra, by its nature and the weight that it occupies within the Hindu and Tantric philosophy, is not only and simply an exercise through which to achieve physical well-being, but it is also a sacred gesture and so it must be approached with full awareness.

General benefits of mudras

Mudras act at the level of subtle energies and each of them has specific qualities that benefit the practitioner in one way or another. For this reason it is difficult to draw up a list of generic benefits of mudras.

It is, however, shown that they, while acting as vehicles of subtle energies that are channeled into our bodies for healing purposes, produce effects on the physical plane.

Each part of the body is in some measure connected to another, and in this sense acting on one side also produces effects on the corresponding part bound to it.

For example, the reflex that is generated by the separation of the fingers of the hands in certain mudras produces a stretching and separation of the dorsal vertebra, which in turn leads to an increase in lung capacity.

The mudras described in this book are particularly indicated to relieve cervical and lumbar pain.

List of body Mudras

Below you will find the description of two body mudras and how to properly execute them. These exercises, combined with yoga asanas, pranayama and relaxation techniques, will be of great benefit to relieve back pain.

Surya Chandra Mudra (Mudra of the Sun and the Moon)

Sitting comfortably with your back straight and your legs crossed (easy pose, Sukasana). The body during this mudra will remain motionless, only the neck will move.

Inhale and, by exhaling, bend the head forward until it touches the sternum with the chin. Inhaling again, rotate the neck to the right to the shoulder. Exhale, return to the initial position. Inhale again and turn the neck to the left. Exhale, return to the initial position. Finally, repeat the exercise in the other direction.

Benefits:

• prevents the cervical

• helps to eliminate headaches

• strengthens the sight

• helps to relax

Contraindications:

• do not practice this mudra in case of arthritis in the cervical vertebrae

Natya Mudra

Sitting in easy position (Sukasana), put the chest out, keep the shoulders back and elbows forward.

This mudra consists of three different phases, to be carried out one after the other without interruption.

First phase: breathing in and out, slightly inflating and deflating the abdomen, imagining that the breath enters and exits the navel. Perform five deep breaths, focusing on abdominal breathing.

Second phase: breathing in, stretching the arms along the sides. Exhale, flex the elbows, bringing out the fingers of the hands with the palms facing up, bringing the wrists as close as possible to the shoulders.

At this point, inhaling and exhaling, opening and closing the ribcage respectively, imagining that the breath enters and comes out of a hole located in the chest. Perform five deep breaths, focusing on chest breathing.

Third phase: breathing in, stretch the arms up, combining the palms of the hands. Exhale and flex your elbows without taking your hands off and touching your head with your wrists.

Imagine that the breath enters and comes out of a hole placed on the throat. Perform five breaths, which will be short and fast.

A final phase, if we can define it, is that of returning to the initial position. Inhale again and lift the arms, exhale and bring them back to the position described in the second step, performing five chest breaths. Inhale again and extend the arms, returning them to the starting position, performing five abdominal breathing.

Benefits:

- stimulates the endorphin system

- revitalizes the body by improving circulation of *prana*

- restores the mind-body connection

Relaxation exercises:

In this chapter we will talk about relaxation exercises. What they are, how they should be performed and what benefits they bring to our psycho-physical health.

These techniques, which will be described in detail below, are a great help to relieve muscular and mental tension and promote the elimination of back pain.

What are relaxation exercises?

When we talk about relaxation in the practice of yoga, we refer concretely to a series of exercises that are normally practiced at the beginning or end (or even in both cases) of a yoga session.

However, this is not just a way to ease the tension or to relax the nerves or even to fall asleep (although these effects are not undesirable and actually happen). In yoga we speak, in relation to this type of exercises, of deep relaxation.

Deep relaxation in yoga is comparable to a state of dynamic sleep that leads to complete relaxation from a physical and mental point of view, encouraging dissolution of muscle tension and helping to reduce stress.

These tensions may be just muscular (due mainly to the assumption of unnatural postures or in the daily execution of certain movements in a wrong way) or mental type (due to excessive mental activity or the constant projection of negative thoughts that arise negative reactions on the physical body).

Without wishing to enter into the details of this vast subject, which would deserve a separate book, it must be said that the body and the mind are strictly bound, to the point that the projection of certain thoughts gives rise to a direct physical effect.

Two opposite examples can be those in which seeing a horror film or an erotic film. In the first case we will probably be experiencing fear or worry, which are reflected in muscular tensions in our body or we might notice how they could for example sweat our hands.

On the contrary, while watching an erotic film it is normal to feel excited and to experiment with other sensations, which can be reflected in much more pleasant physical manifestations.

This is due to the functioning of the autonomic nervous system.

How to practice relaxation exercises

The relaxation exercises that we will see in this book are performed in two positions: lying on the ground or sitting comfortably.

In any case it will always be important to keep the attention placed on the body, so as to eliminate as much as possible any kind of tension, starting from lying down or sitting in a comfortable position, making sure you have a well-aligned back and shoulders not contracted.

Just as in the practice of yoga asanas, it is advisable to wear comfortable clothing, which does not cause discomfort or distractions during practice, even when performing the relaxation exercises.

Moreover, and this is especially true especially in some deep relaxation exercises such as Savasana, it is advisable to cover yourself with a blanket (those who have practiced yoga will know that this is very common), for two different reasons.

From a purely physiological point of view, during body relaxation the body temperature tends to lower, so it is important to keep it constant by covering it with a blanket. From a psychological point of view, cover yourself with a blanket that generates warmth, gives you a sense of comforting security and this helps abandonment and the melting of physical and mental tensions.

It is also important to ensure that you perform these exercises in an environment that promotes relaxation. We will therefore avoid too bright or noisy places (the ideal is to perform the exercises in a space surrounded by silence), preferring those in which there is a pleasant temperature (neither too hot nor too cold) or where we feel at ease.

During the relaxation exercises, pleasant feelings will be felt, such as the dissolving of muscular tensions and pacification of the mind. However, small physical reactions such as chills, tremors, tingling may also occur, usually for very short periods of time.

All this is normal and is yet another demonstration of how body and mind are actually connected, these symptoms being in fact only the manifestation on a physical plane of emotions (often at an unconscious level) that are made to emerge during deep relaxation.

General benefits of relaxation exercises

During deep relaxation, our body experiences organic responses opposite to those produced by stress.

The conscious attention on the body and its "abandonment" during exercise, as well as the awareness of breathing, lead to a state of calm that causes the mind to send signals to the body of absence of danger that manifest themselves underneath form of deep relaxation.

The achievement of this state brings a series of benefits at a physical and mental level, among the main ones we list:

• reduces muscle tension

• relieves pain

• helps reduce anxiety

• reduces stress

• increases awareness

• increases the ability to concentrate

• increases memory

• balances the functioning of the thyroid

• regulates blood pressure

• improves the functioning of the genitourinary apparatus

• improves digestion

• strengthens the immune system

Contraindications:

Although the deep relaxation exercises are mostly safe, in some cases they are not advisable or it is better to perform them under supervision. Although these are not frequent reactions, it is possible that people suffering from dissociative disorders or mental conditions such as paranoia may experience unpleasant feelings due to the way in which these relaxation techniques act on the mind.

List of relaxation exercises

Below you will find a description of two relaxation exercises that we will use in the series of exercises indicated in the next chapter, together with yoga asanas, pranayama techniques and body mudras, with the aim of reducing or eliminating back pain.

Savasana (complete relaxation)

This relaxation exercise is also translated as "position of the corpse", from the Sanskrit "Shava" or cadaver (शव) and "asana" or position (आसन). It goes without saying that the purpose of this exercise is to achieve a deep state of relaxation.

Supine, relax the whole body. Focus on one leg and, inhaling, stretch all the muscles. Exhale slowly and deeply, relax the foot, ankle, calf, knee, thigh and gluteus, until the entire leg is completely relaxed. Proceed by performing the same procedure with the other leg.

At this point concentrate on the torso, inhaling and exhaling slowly and progressively relaxing each part, starting from the hips, abdomen, chest and shoulders, until you feel that this part of the body is completely relaxed.

Focus now on one arm. Inhaling, tighten the fist and stretch all the muscles. Exhale, relax the hand, the wrist, the forearm, the elbow, the arm and the shoulder. Perform the same procedure on the other arm.

Focus now on your neck and throat, relaxing by inhaling and exhaling.

Continue with your face. Keep eyes and lips slightly ajar, inhale and exhale, relaxing lips, chin, cheeks, ears, nose, eyes, forehead and head.

Stay still for a few minutes, listening to your breathing and feeling the total relaxation of the body.

Before lifting, roll the body gently in one direction and another.

Benefits:

• reduces stress and nervous tension

• reduces muscle tension

• improves concentration

• helps to fight insomnia

• relaxes the muscles

• calms the mind

• stimulates circulation

Shoulder relaxation exercise

This exercise can be performed on your feet or on your knees, keeping your torso upright, your arms relaxed and your eyes closed.

Focus on one shoulder: inhale and lift it with a slow, circular motion. Exhale, lower it. Each phase of breathing (both inhalation and exhalation) must last approximately five seconds.

Repeat the exercise three times with one shoulder, then change shoulder and repeat in the same way.

Eventually you can perform the exercise with the two shoulders at the same time, making them rotate slowly forward and backward, inhaling in the thrust movement of the shoulders upward and exhaling in the movement that brings the shoulders down.

Benefits:

• reduces muscle tension

Set of exercises for back pain

The corrective exercises proposed in this chapter are aimed at reversing bad posture and generally improving the level of well-being of the skeletal and muscular system, eliminating back pain.

Anyone suffering from lateral curvature of the spine (scoliosis), curvature of the spine in the thoracic or sacral region (kyphosis), cervical, lumbar or dorsal arthritis will be able to benefit greatly from these exercises, provided they are performed in the correct manner that has been explained above.

These are just some examples of series of exercises that can be combined to solve some more advanced medical situations, using some of the exercises presented earlier in the book (asanas, mudras, pranayamas and relaxation exercises).

I urge you to try the various exercises always with caution and paying the utmost attention to the sensations of your body, trying to dissolve the tensions with the proposed relaxation exercises and in general by using these exercises as an instrument of self-knowledge.

Exercises for lumbar and back pain

The following two sets of exercises have been studied to prevent and treat pain in the dorsal and lumbar region of the back.

Perform the exercises as explained in the previous chapters, keeping the attention on your body and trying to achieve them in the absence of effort and in a conscious state.

First set of exercises

- Dharmikasana (devotional pose)

- Dandasana (stick pose)

- Anantasana (side-reclining leg lift pose)

- Setu Bandhasana (bridge pose)

- Ganapatiasana (Ganesha pose)

- Chatushkonasana (position of the square)

- Trikonasana (triangle pose)

- Sayana Buddhasana (reclining Buddha pose)

- Surya Chandra Pranayama

- Savasana (complete relaxation)

Second set of exercises

- Surya Namaskara (sun salutation)

- Dandasana (stick pose)

- Anantadana (side-reclining leg lift pose)

- Supta Konasana (reclining bound angle pose)

- Setu Bandhasana (bridge pose)

- Trikonasana (triangle pose)

- Sayana Buddhasana (reclining Buddha pose)

- Surya Chandra Pranayama

- Surya Chandra Mudra

- Savasana (complete relaxation)

Exercises for cervical pain

The following two sets of exercises have been studied to prevent and treat pain in the neck and neck area.

Pay particular attention to the movements of your body, make sure they are not brusque and if you notice that you feel nauseous or have the feeling that your head was spinning, stop the exercises and concentrate on breathing, keeping calm.

This is a normal reaction (which will not necessarily appear), but which will tend to present itself less and less with practice.

First set of exercises

• Shoulder relaxation

• Ardha Bhujangasana (half cobra pose)

• Setu Bandhasana (bridge pose)

• Surya Chandra Pranayama

• Natya Mudra

• Complete yogic breathing

• Savasana (complete relaxation)

Second set of exercises

- Surya Namaskara (sun salutation)

- Ardha Chandrasana (half-moon pose)

- Setu Bandhasana (bridge pose)

- Surya Chandra Pranayama

- Surya Chandra Mudra

- Natya Mudra

- Savasana (complete relaxation)

Exercises for the lateral curvature of the column (scoliosis)

The following two sets of exercises have been studied to correct scoliosis and in general the curvatures of the spine, which can generate atrophy or muscle hypertrophy.

First set of exercises

- Surya Namaskara (sun salutation)

- Anjaneyasana (low lunge pose)

- Ardha Chandrasana (half-moon pose)

- Natarajasana (lord of the dance pose)

- Complete yogic breathing

- Savasana (complete relaxation)

Second set of exercises

- Surya Namaskara (sun salutation)

- Sadhakasana (pose of the adept)

- Dandasana (stick pose)

- Trikonasana (triangle pose)

- Parivrtta Trikonasana (revolved triangle pose)

- Complete yogic breathing

- Savasana (complete relaxation)

Exercises for the curvature of the spine in the thoracic or sacral region (kyphosis)

The following two sets of exercises have been studied to correct the curvature of the spine in the thoracic or sacral area, also known as kyphosis.

In the case of kyphosis, even mild, it is important to try to correct the posture of the spine, since any increase in the curvature could lead to suffering from arthritis in the future.

First set of exercises

- Sadhakasana (pose of the adept)

- Bhujangasana (cobra pose)

- Ganapatiasana (Ganesha pose)

- Tadasana (mountain pose)

- Ardha Natyasana (half dance pose)

- Surya Chandra Pranayama

- Complete yogic breathing

- Savasana (complete relaxation)

Second set of exercises

- Surya Namaskara (sun salutation)
- Setu Bandhasana (bridge pose)
- Dhanurasana (bow pose)
- Ganapatiasana (Ganesha pose)
- Tadasana (mountain pose)
- Ardha Natyasana (half dance pose)
- Complete yogic breathing
- Surya Chandra Pranayama
- Savasana (complete relaxation)

Basic Sanskrit glossary

The table below shows a number of basic Sanskrit terms that you can meet in this book, with the corresponding English translation.

English	Sanskrit	Meaning
Adho	अधो	downward
Ardha	अर्ध	half
Asana	आसन	posture, seat
Bandha	बंध	lock
Dhánus	धनुः	bow
Dvī	द्वि	two
Eka	एक	one, single
Guru	गुरू	master, teacher, guide
Mantra	मन्त्र	from the union of the verb root "man" (thinking) and the suffix "between" (which protects)
Mudra	मुद्रा	seal, gesture
Parivṛtta	परिवृत्त	revolved, twisted
Parsva	पार्श्व	side, flank
Prana	प्राण	life force, vital principle
Sukha	सुख	pleasure
Supta	सुप्त	supine
		reclining
Tana	तान	stretched

Tulā	तुला	balance
Ud	उद्	prefix for verbs or nouns, indicating superiority in location, rank, power, intensity
Upaviṣṭha	उपवष्िठ	seated
Ubhaya	उभय	both, together
Ūrdhva	ऊर्ध्व	upward
Uttana	उत्तान	intense stretch
Utthita	उत्थति	extended